ATKINS DIET COOKBOOK

Best Low Carb Recipes to Burn Your Fat

DEBORAH SWAN

Contents

Introduction

You have probably heard about the Atkins Diet, but do you know that much about it? You might also have a negative mindset towards this diet, having heard rumors about it in the past, but the bottom line is that everything changes over time, and that includes the Atkins Diet.

Put simply, the Atkins diet is a very effective and easy to follow diet, one which gives you guaranteed, effective results, and also helps you learn and recognize healthy food habits which will change your outlook on dietary nutrition for life.

No counting, no red or green days, and nothing too complicated in the slightest.

If you have picked up this book then you are no doubt very interested in following the Atkins Diet, and you have probably already learned a little about it to start with. At first, we will reiterate the diet's history, how it works, how to follow it, and also quickly run through the phases and what you need to do in each one. After that, we will get onto the practical stuff, the recipes!

The aim of this book is to show you that the Atkins Diet gives you endless choice and freedom when it comes to delicious meals and snacks. You don't have to be a super chef to be able to follow this diet, and you don't need to spend a fortune on expensive ingredients – many ingredients for this diet are already in your fridge, freezer, or kitchen cupboards.

So, let's get onto the mechanics of the diet, before moving onto the recipes themselves.

All About The Atkins Diet

Diets are generally not fun, they cause hunger, headaches, stress, and you basically get so annoyed at the fact the scales aren't moving as fast as you would like them to, that you give up entirely. What does this do? Totally erodes at your self-esteem, and does nothing for your waistline.

The chances are that you have tried many different diets in the past, and if you have got to this point and you're picking this book up, the chances also are that those other diets didn't work. Never fear however, because the Atkins Diet is proven to be highly effective, and it also helps you understand nutrition in a totally different way.

What is The Atkins Diet?

The Atkins Diet is a low carbohydrate diet, which limits the amount of carbohydrates you eat per day, and instead focuses your attention on proteins and fats. You might think that fats are bad, but the science really explains it.

Regular diets focus on low calorie, high carbohydrate intake. When you limit the amount of calories you are eating, your body begins to burn the carbohydrates for fuel, e.g. the energy you need to go about your daily business, and it stockpiles fats, because it basically thinks it's not going to get anymore. Now, if you have a lot of weight to lose, the fact that your body's fuel burning system isn't touching those fat stores, really doesn't do much for your waistline. What you want to do is to eat into those fat stores, which is what happens when you go onto a low carbohydrate diet.

When you limit the amount of carbohydrates you are eating, your body is forced to think and act in a different way, e.g. it has to burn fats for fuel, rather than carbs, and that means it is effectively eating into those fat stores you are so badly wanting to get rid of.

Bingo!

Now, in order for your body to change its way of thinking, it has to kickstart a normal metabolic process called ketosis.

What is Ketosis?

Don't worry about this rather scary, scientific name, because ketosis is actually something your body does perfectly naturally, and it isn't dangerous at all.

Ketosis is often linked with diabetes treatment, but that doesn't mean that by forcing your body to work with ketosis that you are diabetic, or that you have any risk in the slightest; in actual fact, ketosis and weight loss work together very well indeed. When you are following the Atkins Diet, you are forcing your body into this state in the first phase, and then after that you are slowly removing yourself from it, until you reach a natural level where your body is able to stay at a steady weight level.

When your body begins to burn fat for energy, as you are doing when you begin the Atkins diet, it begins to produce ketones. Now, this isn't harmful, but the most important thing is that you need to keep your protein levels at the recommended amount, to stop any adverse effects – provided you do that, there is no need to worry, and no concerns required. Ketosis is basically that you are changing the way your body works in terms of burning fuel for energy, and that's all you really need to know.

The History of the Atkins Diet

The Atkins Diet was developed by Dr Robert Akins, an American cardiologist, who learned that low carbohydrate diets not only helped his client with their heart issues, but also helped them lose considerable amounts of weight too. Obviously when a person has heart problems and is obese too, this does not help the initial issue, so weight loss in turn did wonders for his patients.

Over time the diet has undergone many changes, originally being quite hard to follow, but now it has changed to something much easier, and provided you read the guidelines and understand the science behind the diet, you will be able to fit it all into your day without having to give it too much thought.

The Advantages of the Atkins Diet

- It gives you guaranteed weight loss
- It allows you to consider nutritional options
- It makes you think about your health and be more mindful about your choices
- It is easy to follow
- You can switch back to the beginning once you have completed the final phase, if you find any weight is creeping back on
- You can basically eat until you are full, without having to stop because of calories or portion control
- You can eat the foods you can't on other diets, e.g. high fat foods
- Only the first phase is particularly restrictive, but even that is quite generous
- There are many recipes you can follow and many foods you can eat
- You will not get hungry
- You won't get cravings

The Phases of the Atkins Diet

What sets the Atkins Diet apart from other low carb diets, such as the Paleo or the Keto Diet is that it has set phases which are distinctly different from each other. To give you a basis run down, because by picking up this book we are assuming you already know a little about the diet, and we are going to give a more in-depth description as we talk about recipes for each phase:

Phase 1 – Induction Stage

This is the most restrictive stage of the diet, and during this particular phase it is important to not go over your carbohydrate intake limit, which is 20g per day; having said that, you shouldn't go under 18g, because you need a set amount for you body to function healthily.

In this stage you are forcing your body into ketosis, so this is when you are more likely to notice side effects, however most of these can be side-stepped or at least minimized by eating more salt and drinking plenty of water. At this stage however, you should learn to read food labels quite well, because there are many hidden carbs out there which can impact your diet if you aren't aware of them.

This particular phase generally lasts for 2 weeks and is the part where you lose the most drastic amount of weight. It is possible to stay in this phase for a little longer, but this is a personal decision, depending on how much weight you have to lose.

Phase 2 – Food Induction Stage

In this second stage you need to gradually increase the number of carbs you have in your diet, to no more than 25g. This obviously means you have slightly more freedom in terms of what you can and can't eat, but you should still remain mindful. This particular phase is about slowly slowly moving towards your maintenance phase, and again, you can decide how long you stay in this phase.

Phase 3 – Ongoing Weight Loss Stage

The ongoing trend of slowly introducing more carbs into your diet begins in phase three. The aim of this particular phase is that you will have reached your goal by the end of it, so you should keep an eye on the scales at this point. In this phase you are allowed a total daily carbohydrate allowance of 35g.

Phase 4 - Maintenance Stage

This isn't really a phase because it is the food pattern and lifestyle choice for the rest of your days. Basically you have reached your goal at this point, and you should be congratulated! Here you find your natural carb allowance, the point where your body maintains a natural weight, without increasing or decreasing.

If you find you are putting a little weight back on, this is the point where you can play around with your carb allowance slightly, dropping it by 5g and seeing how you go, before increasing back up for a time – this about trial and error to a degree, but generally speaking, by this point you are very aware of your nutritional choices, and you are feeling healthier as a result.

Your Path to Great Health And a Slimmer Waistline

When you choose to follow the Atkins Diet, you are joining countless others who have all chosen the same path and have successfully lost the weight they wanted to aim towards, and have kept it off too.

Of course, the most important thing to remember is that you need to put the effort in to get anything out, and that means mixing your meals up to avoid boredom. Probably the biggest advantage of going down the Atkins Diet route is that you don't get hungry, and with some of the easy recipes we're going to describe in this book, you will be ready and raring to go!

So, without further ado, let's check out the delicious meals you can eat in each phase of the Atkins Diet.

2

Recipes For The Atkins Diet
Phase 1

Quick Reminder of Phase 1

Phase 1 is the starting point of your Atkins Diet journey, and this is where you are restricting your carbohydrate intake the most. Having said that, there is a lot of scope for what you can eat at this point, so it isn't as restrictive as some regular low-calorie diets you may have tried in the past.

This is the stage where you may get more in the way of side effects, because you are forcing your body into a different way of thinking, e.g. ketosis, and that means you are in a transitional period, whilst your body gets used to this new way of thinking. Many of these issues, such as headaches and sleep disturbances, can be overcome by making sure you stay hydrated and drink enough water, and also by adding salt to basically everything; this is all down to mineral loss, and by drinking water and adding salt, you are replacing what you aren't getting. This is also the phase where you may find you end up going to the toilet to pee a little more, because your body is releasing water stores by going into ketosis – simply make sure you stay hydrated and don't be too far from the toilet!

- Do not eat more than 22g of carbs per day, but don't go under 18g. The general figure at this stage is 20g
- This phase lasts for an average of 2 weeks, but this is a personal decision
- You will lose the most weight during this stage
- Ensure you eat 4-6oz of protein per day, depending on your body weight, and adjust accordingly as you lose weight

Baked Meatballs

Cooking time: Half an hour
Recipe makes 4 servings
Total carbs per serving 1.8g

Ingredients

- Extra virgin olive oil, 1 tablespoon
- Spring onion
- Garlic, 1.5 teaspoons
- Ground veal, 0.5lb
- Ground beef, 0.5lb
- Ground pork, 0.5lb
- Granted parmesan cheese, 0.5 cup
- 2 large eggs

- Salt, 0.5 teaspoon
- Black pepper, 0.25 teaspoon

Method

1. Pre-heat the oven to 190°C
2. Cook the onion until soft
3. Add the garlic to the onion and cook for one minute extra
4. In a large bowl, combine the veal, beef, and pork
5. Add into the bowl the rest of the ingredients and mix well
6. Roll into small meatballs and place on a baking tray
7. Bake in the oven for 25 minutes, until cooked

Tips & Tricks/Did You Know?

You might have this particular dish down as a dinner recipe, but it is actually a breakfast dish, which goes very well to start your day! The filling nature of this dish will keep you full and also works a part of your protein intake.

Egg Salad

Cooking time: Less than 5 minutes
Recipe makes 4 servings
Total carbs per serving 2.4g

Ingredients

- Boiled eggs, around 8

- Full mayonnaise, 0.5 cup
- Dijon mustard, 3 tablespoons
- 0.5 teaspoon of salt
- 0.25 teaspoon of black pepper
- Celery stalks, around 2 will be enough

Method

1. Boil the eggs as usual, to your liking
2. Chop the boiled eggs up into rough or small pieces, depending on how you like them
3. Mix the eggs together with the mayonnaise, the mustard, and the salt and pepper
4. Combine well
5. Chop up the celery into small pieces and add to the mixture
6. You can now serve the mixture, lettuce is a good serving bed

Tips & Tricks/Did You Know?

This particular dish is not only for phase 1 because you can have this at any phase and add in low carb bread or a tortilla, as you add more carbs to your diet in the next few phases. Remember to adjust the carb amount by doing this.

Asparagus with sun-dried tomato vinaigrette

Cooking time: Less than 5 minutes
Recipe makes 6 servings
Total carbs per serving 3.2g

Ingredients

- Asparagus spears, around 30 in total
- Sun-dried tomatoes, 1.5oz
- 1 tablespoon of balsamic vinegar
- 1 tablespoon of red wine vinegar
- Garlic – ¼ teaspoon
- 3 tablespoons of extra virgin olive oil

Method

1. Place the asparagus in a steamer, or place over a steaming pot of boiling water for around 4 minutes, covered over. Ensure the asparagus is tender and green before removing from the heat.
2. Add the rest of the ingredients into a blender and combine
3. Add salt and pepper to taste
4. Drizzle on top of the asparagus and serve

Tips & Tricks/Did You Know?

To ensure the asparagus is properly cooked, you should let it stay on the heat until it is bright green and tender, not at all crispy. Red wine vinegar is also best as it is less acidic than regular vinegar, and works very well with the balsamic for an extra luxurious taste!

Breakfast Muffins

Cooking time: Half an hour
Recipe makes 6 servings

Total carbs per serving 1.4g

Ingredients

- Choose between bacon, ham, or sausage, 1lb of either, broken into small pieces
- Shredded cheese, 8oz
- 4 eggs
- Heavy cream, 1.5 cups

Method

1. Preheat the oven to 200°C
2. Take a large muffin tray and spray it with non-stick spray
3. Divide the meat into each muffin tray section
4. Add cheese equally into each section
5. In a bowl, mix together the eggs and heavy cream
6. Pour this mixture over each section
7. Bake for half an hour, until golden and spongy

Tips & Tricks/Did You Know?

If you're looking for a bakery-style treat in the morning, or perhaps a snack or lunch time pick me up, this is an ideal dish to try. Bake them in the morning or the night before, let them cool and store them in a plastic tub, taking them to work with you, and getting you through the day.

Broccoli & Cauliflower Cheese Bake

Cooking time: 20 minutes

Recipe makes 6 servings
Total carbs per serving 8.5g

Ingredients

- 3 large broccoli – chopped
- 2 large cauliflower – chopped
- Jar of pimentos, 2 tablespoons
- Half a yellow bell pepper – chopped
- Ricotta cheese, 0.5 cup
- Non fat cottage cheese, 1 cup
- Shredded cheddar, 1 cup
- Skimmed mozzarella, shredded, 3oz

Method

1. Preheat the oven to 160°C
2. In a large bowl, combine all ingredients
3. Take a casserole dish/pan and spray with non-stick spray, place the mixture inside the dish/pan
4. Bake in the oven for 15 minutes

Tips & Tricks/Did You Know?

The high fat content of this dish is ideal for the first phase of the Atkins diet, and this is also one of the most filling dishes you can have. This particular dish is ideal for an evening meal, and will also give you a good protein hit, at 15.2g per serving.

Beef Chili Stroganoff

Cooking time: Half an hour
Recipe makes 2 servings
Total carbs per serving 13.4g

Ingredients

- Brussel sprouts, around 10
- Brown mushrooms, 6oz
- Olive oil, 2 tablespoons
- Thyme, 2 teaspoons
- Paprika, 1 teaspoon
- Cinnamon, 1/8 teaspoon
- Garlic, 2 cloves
- Ground beef, 14oz
- Chili powder, 1 tablespoon
- Salt, 1 teaspoon
- Black pepper, 0.5 teaspoon
- Tomato paste, 2 tablespoons
- Sour cream, 0.25 cup

Method

1. Place a pot of water on the stove and bring it to the boil
2. Cut the Brussel sprouts in half and add them to the boiling water
3. Over a medium to high heat, add the oil to a skillet pan and allow to warm up
4. Chop up the mushrooms whilst the pan is heating up
5. Add the mushrooms to the pan and cook for just over 5 minutes, until brown

6. To the pan, add the thyme, paprika, cinnamon, and garlic and cook for half a minute more – keep stirring
7. Remove the Brussel sprouts from the heat and drain
8. Place the sprouts into serving plates
9. Heat up the ground beef, seasoning with the chili powder, salt, and pepper until brown
10. Add the tomato paste to the beef pan and cook for a further 3 minutes
11. Add the sour cream and stir in, cooking until beginning to bubble
12. Serve the mixture over the sprouts

Tips & Tricks/Did You Know?

This particular dish is ideal for a hearty evening meal, and is a great twist on the classic stroganoff recipe. By using Brussel sprouts you are getting your serving of vitamins, and the luxurious taste of the cream and beef together will certainly have you wanting to cook it again!

Bratwurst With Sauerkraut

Cooking time: 10 minutes
Recipe makes 1 serving
Total carbs per serving 3.6g

Ingredients

- 1 Bratwurst, around 3oz in weight
- Canned sauerkraut, 0.5 cup

Method

1. Preheat a grill to a medium to high heat
2. Grill the bratwurst until browned all over, turning regularly
3. Alternatively, you can microwave the bratwurst for 1-2 minutes
4. Remove the sauerkraut from the can and heat up in microwave oven
5. Serve together whilst warm

Tips & Tricks/Did You Know?

This particular dish is a popular German favorite, whilst also being filling and nutritious for phase 1 of the Atkins Diet. You can easily find both ingredients in supermarkets, and this dish is also a good source of protein, containing 12.3g per serving.

Browned Pumpkin With Maple & Sage

Cooking time: 10 minutes
Recipe makes 8 servings
Total carbs per serving 3.5g

Ingredients

- Pumpkin, 1lb
- Shallots, chopped, 0.25 cup
- Unsalted butter, 1 tablespoon
- Vegetable broth, 0.25 cup
- Sugar free syrup, 1/16 cup

- Ground sage, 0.25 teaspoon

Method

1. Over a medium to high heat, melt the butter in a skillet pan
2. Cut the pumpkin into chunks, around ¾"
3. Add the pumpkin and the shallots to the pan
4. Season with salt and black pepper
5. Cook until pumpkin has browned and the shallots are clear, this should take just over 5 minutes
6. Turn down the heat and add the vegetable broth
7. Cover the pan and simmer for 10 minutes, or until the pumpkin is tender
8. Add the maple syrup and the sage, stirring everything together
9. Serve

Tips & Tricks/Did You Know?

To give extra taste and luxury to this particular recipe, use fresh sage, rather than anything else. Around 7/8 leaves will be enough.

Crustless Quiche

Cooking time: 95 minutes
Recipe makes 8 servings
Total carbs per serving 4.7g

Ingredients

- Bacon, 4oz
- Half an onion, sliced
- 6 eggs
- Heavy cream, 0.75 cup
- Broccoli or spinach, 10oz each
- Shredded Swiss cheese, 0.5lb
- Salt, 0.5 teaspoon
- Pepper 0.25 teaspoon

Method

1. Preheat the oven to 180°C
2. Take a 10" quiche pan or a 9" deep pan, butter it to avoid sticking
3. In a skillet pan, cook the bacon until crisp
4. Chop once cooked
5. Remove the oil from the bacon pan, keeping 1 tablespoon of it aside
6. Add the onions to the pan and cook for around 5 minutes, combining with the bacon oil
7. Combine the eggs, cream, broccoli, cheese, salt, and pepper into a large bowl
8. Stir in the bacon and onion
9. Pour the whole mixture into the oiled pan
10. Bake in the oven for around 1 hour and 15 minutes, until cooked
11. Allow to cool before cutting into slices

Tips & Tricks/Did You Know?

This is a great recipe for preparing ahead, e.g. for work lunches or even party food. Keep your quiche chilled in the fridge, allowing it to totally cook beforehand, and whip it out when you want to pack your lunch, or you need a snack!

Buffalo Chicken Salad

Cooking time: 45 minutes
Recipe makes 2 servings
Total carbs per serving 9.7g

Ingredients

- Half a lemon
- 1 medium young green onion
- 1 head of Romaine or cos lettuce
- 2 medium celery stalks
- 1 red sweet pepper
- 1 tomato, medium
- 1 egg
- Apple cider vinegar, 5 1/3 tablespoons
- Celery salt, 1/8 teaspoons
- Cayenne pepper, 1/8 teaspoons
- Chicken thighs with bone removed, x 2
- Mayonnaise, 0.25 cup
- Sour cream, 2 tablespoons
- Blue cheese 2 or 3 oz
- Garlic powder 1/8 teaspoons
- Salt, 1/3 teaspoons
- Black pepper, ¼ teaspoons

Method

1. Preheat the oven to 230°C

2. Remove the juice from the lemon into a bowl
3. Chop up the greens finely and add them to the bowl
4. Add the mayonnaise, sour cream, blue cheese, and garlic powder, stirring to combine together
5. Cut up the lettuce and add to the dressing
6. Cut the celery into small pieces and add to the dressing also
7. Cut up the bell pepper and tomato and add to the bowl
8. Put the bowl into the fridge
9. Beat the eggs together and add the apple cider vinegar black pepper, salt, celery salt, and cayenne pepper – stir together well
10. Add the chicken to the marinade and bake for 20 minutes, turning and re-brushing a few times. The chicken is cooked when it is crisp
11. Cut up the chicken and set aside
12. Take the salad from the fridge and toss
13. Add the chicken and serve

Tips & Tricks/Did You Know?

If you love chicken Caesar salad, this is actually a good alternative twist for the first phase of your Atkins journey, whilst having plenty of spicy kick! This works best as a lunchtime treat.

Buttermilk Cinnamon Waffles

Cooking time: 15 minutes
Recipe makes 8 servings

Total carbs per serving 5.4g

Ingredients

- Whole grain soy flour, 1 cup
- Sugar substitute sweetener, 2 tablespoons
- Cinnamon, 2 teaspoons
- Baking powder, 3 teaspoons
- Baking soda, 0.5 teaspoons
- Buttermilk, 0.75 cup
- Unsalted butter, 6 tablespoons
- 3 large eggs
- Sugar free vanilla syrup, 1.5oz
- Tap water, 0.5 cup
- Cooking spray

Method

1. Heat up the waffle pan
2. Add together the soy flour, sugar substitute, cinnamon, baking powder, and soda
3. Add the buttermilk, butter, eggs, and syrup to the mixture and stir well
4. Add the cold water gradually to the mixture, 1 tablespoon at a time; the batter should resemble a pancake batter
5. Spray the waffle pan with cooking spray
6. Add the batter to the waffle pan and cook until crisp and brown
7. Repeat the process until the batter has gone

Tips & Tricks/Did You Know?

This American style breakfast treat gives you a 6.9g boost of protein to start your day. You might think that finding the buttermilk could be difficult, but check your supermarket shelves and you will surely find it! You will need a waffle pan for this particular recipe.

Buttered Brussel Sprouts

Cooking time: 10 minutes
Recipe makes 4 servings
Total carbs per serving 2.3g

Ingredients

- Brussel sprouts, 2 cups
- Unsalted butter, 2 tablespoons

Method

1. Trim the Brussel sprouts and cut them into halves
2. Salt and boil water and cook the sprouts for around 8 minutes, until they are tender
3. Drain the sprouts
4. Melt the butter over a medium heat
5. Add the sprouts and toss, ensuring they are fully coated
6. Season with salt and pepper

Tips & Tricks/Did You Know?

Adding nutmeg to the sprouts gives the dish a different kind of taste. If you're not a big fan of sprouts, try them this way, you will be converted!

Cheddar Omelet with Sautéed Onions

Cooking time: 15 minutes
Recipe makes 1 servings
Total carbs per serving 6.8g

Ingredients

- Chopped onions, 1/3 cup
- Extra virgin olive oil, 1 tablespoon
- Shredded cheddar cheese, 0.5 cup
- 2 eggs
- 1 sliced scallion

Method

1. Sauté the onions in olive oil until translucent
2. Remove from the pan and set to one side
3. Beat the eggs and add to the same pan
4. Cook until they begin to bubble, before flipping over
5. Add the cheese, onions and scallions to this side and cook for a further minute
6. Fold the omelette in half and cook for a further minute
7. Season to taste

Tips & Tricks/Did You Know?

The omelet is a classic breakfast dish, but can actually be enjoyed at any time of the day. The great thing about this particular dish is that because of the eggs and cheese content, it gives you a big protein hit to start your day, if you choose it for breakfast.

3

Recipes For The Atkins Diet
Phase 2

Quick Reminder of Phase 2

Phase 2 is where you are going to slowly introduce more carbohydrates into your diet, but in a slow and steady manner. At this phase you should be over halfway to your final goal, and your food choices can be a little greater now you are moving towards the end of your weight loss aims. Because your body is still in ketosis, this is the phase where you probably need to be the most careful in terms of checking the scales, but do not do this every day, as your body does fluctuate naturally – once per week is enough.

- Eat 25g of carbohydrates per day
- Remember to stick to your protein allowance
- You can remain in phase 2 for as long as you want to, but then move onto phase 3

Artichokes With Lemon Butter

Cooking time: 25 minutes
Recipe makes 4 servings
Total carbs per serving 9.9g

Ingredients

- Medium artichokes, x 4
- Lemons x 4
- Coriander seed, 2 tablespoons
- Salt, 2 tablespoons
- Unsalted butter, 0.5 cup

Method

1. Bring some water to the boil
2. Trim and cut the artichokes and boil
3. Cut 3 lemons into halves and squeeze out the juice into some water
4. Add the rest of the lemon halves, coriander seeds, and the salt
5. Place the artichokes into the liquid and cover it over to stop the artichokes from lifting and floating
6. Boil for 15 minutes
7. Remove and drain the water
8. In a small bowl, melt the butter and mix in the juice of the remaining lemon, adding salt and pepper
9. Serve

Tips & Tricks/Did You Know?

This quick and easy dish can be a snack or a meal, the

choice is yours! Whatever you choose, you get a 4.8g hit of protein from chowing down.

Atkins Yorkshire Pudding

Cooking time: 40 minutes
Recipe makes 9 servings
Total carbs per serving 3.8g

Ingredients

- Whole grain soy flour, 0.5 cup
- Wheat gluten, 2oz
- 3 large eggs
- Whole milk, 1 cup
- Salt, 1 teaspoon
- Canola vegetable oil, 1/3 cup
- Baking powder, 1 teaspoon

Method

1. Preheat the oven to 230°C
2. In a small bowl, whisk together the soy flour, gluten, eggs, milk, and the salt, until well combined
3. Prepare a square baking dish with oil
4. Place the dish or tray into the oven for 5 minutes to heat up
5. Add the batter evenly to the dish or tray
6. Bake for 15 minutes
7. Turn the oven down to 170°C and continue to bake for another 15-20 minutes, until the pudding is browned

8. Serve hot

Tips & Tricks/Did You Know?

The Yorkshire pudding is an iconic food type which is often served with Sunday roasts. As you can see, you don't need to sacrifice your Sunday meal for your diet, provided you keep an eye on the carb intake of the rest of your roast ingredients. The pudding itself will give you 9.2g of your protein hit.

Almond Raspberry Cupcakes

Cooking time: 50 minutes
Recipe makes 10 servings
Total carbs per serving 4.8g

Ingredients

- 2 eggs
- Unsalted butter, 0.75 cup
- Sugar substitute, 1/3 cup
- Heavy cream, 2 tablespoons
- Tap water, 1 fluid oz
- Lemon juice, 0.5 teaspoon
- Vanilla extract, 1 teaspoon
- Pure almond extract, 2 teaspoons
- Almond meal flour, 2.5 cups
- Baking powder, 0.5 teaspoons
- Salt, 0.5 teaspoons
- Sugar free red raspberry preserve, 3 1/3 tablespoons

Method

1. Preheat the oven to 230°C
2. In a muffin pan, place muffin cups
3. Beat the egg yolks in a small pan, adding a ¼ cup of sugar substitute, the butter, cream, water, lemon juice and extracts until combined
4. In another bowl, beat the egg whites until they are frothy
5. Add the rest of the sugar substitute and beat until soft peaks have formed
6. Fold the egg whites into the mixture carefully
7. In another bowl still, combine the almond meal, baking powder, and the salt
8. Fold this into the egg mixture and divide between the muffin cups
9. Drop 1 teaspoon of jam into the center of each mixture
10. Bake for half an hour
11. Cool for 20 minutes

Tips & Tricks/Did You Know?

These tasty snacks can be kept for other days, provided you keep them in an airtight container once they have been cooled. They will keep for up to one week.

Beef Huevos Rancheros on Canadian Bacon

Cooking time: 30 minutes
Recipe makes 4 servings
Total carbs per serving 2.5g

Ingredients

- Ground beef, 6 oz
- Green chili peppers, 0.5 cup
- Garlic powder, 0.25 teaspoon
- Chili powder, 1 teaspoon
- Cumin, 0.25 teaspoon
- Oregano, 0.25 teaspoon
- Salt, 0.25 teaspoon
- Black pepper, 0.25 teaspoon
- Canadian bacon, 4 slices
- 4 eggs
- Shredded cheddar cheese, 0.5 cup
- Cilantro, 4 pieces

Method

1. Grease a skillet pan and place on medium heat
2. Add the beef and brown it
3. Add the chilies, garlic, chili powder, cumin, oregano, salt, and pepper. Cook for around 10 minutes
4. Add the bacon over the top of the beef for a few minutes
5. Remove the pan from the heat
6. Heat up another skillet pan with oil and scramble the eggs to your liking
7. To serve, add a piece of bacon to each plate, add some of the beef, and some of the eggs
8. Sprinkle cheese and cilantro on top of the dish

Tips & Tricks/Did You Know?

You can mix this recipe up a little if you prefer a different type of egg, so if you like fried or poached eggs, simply change the way you cook the eggs accordingly.

Grilled Steak With Spicy Salsa

Cooking time: 1 hour
Recipe makes 4 servings
Total carbs per serving 7g

Ingredients

- Ground cumin, 2 tablespoons
- Minced garlic, 3 cloves
- Lime juice, 3 tablespoons
- Black pepper, 1 teaspoon
- Salt, 0.5 teaspoon
- 1 – 1.5lb steak
- 1 chopped tomato
- Mild green chilies, 1 can drained
- 2 sliced scallions
- Chili powder, 0.5 teaspoon

Method

1. Preheat the grill and spray your cooking plate with cooking oil or spray
2. Cook the cumin for around 3 minutes on the skillet
3. Placed the cooked cumin in a small bowl
4. Add the garlic, 2 tablespoons of the lime juice, the black pepper, and ¼ teaspoons of salt. Mix together well

5. Wash the steak and rub the cumin mixture all over
6. Grill the steak and cook to your liking
7. Mix together the tomato, chilies, scallions, chili powder, and the rest of the lime juice and salt
8. Slice the steak and serve with salsa

Tips & Tricks/Did You Know?

Flank steak or top round steak works best for this type of recipe, however if you prefer a different cut you can easily adapt it to your liking.

Bell Pepper Rings Filled With Eggs and Mozzarella

Cooking time: 20 minutes
Recipe makes 1 servings
Total carbs per serving 5.1g

Ingredients

- Sweet red peppers, 1 or 2
- 2 eggs
- Canola vegetable oil, 1 teaspoon
- Shredded mozzarella cheese, 0.25 cup

Method

1. Cut the bell pepper in the middle and cut into rings, removing the seeds
2. Place the rings into the sauté pan over a medium to high heat

3. Add an egg to each ring and cook until done to your liking
4. Add cheese on top of the eggs
5. Cover the pan and cook for a further minute
6. Season with salt and pepper

Tips & Tricks/Did You Know?

By eating this particular recipe you are getting a big intake of antioxidants, so make sure you pick the brightest peppers you can find, to get the most benefit for your health.

Beef Burger With Feta And Tomato

Cooking time: 22 minutes
Recipe makes 4 servings
Total carbs per serving 1.3g

Ingredients

- Ground beef, 1lb
- Spring onion or scallions, one
- Baby spinach, 0.5 cup
- Sliced or chopped tomatoes, 0.25 cup
- Crumbled feta cheese, 0.25 cup
- Fresh dill, 1.5 teaspoons
- Salt, 0.5 teaspoon
- Black pepper, 0.5 teaspoon

Method

1. In a large bowl, mix together with beef, spring onion/scallion, tomato, feta, dill, salt and pepper
2. Split the mixture into four and form burgers
3. Heat a grill or pan to medium heat
4. Cook the burgers on each side for around 6 minutes, or a little more if you prefer well-done burgers

Tips & Tricks/Did You Know?

This particular dish will give you a large hit of your daily protein amount, at 24.3g. You can add in low carb bread if you like a traditional burger, but remember to add the carb amount to your daily allowance.

Almond Protein Pancakes

Cooking time: 15 minutes
Recipe makes 4 servings
Total carbs per serving 4.4g

Ingredients

- Vanilla whey protein, 2oz
- Almond meal flour, 0.25 cup
- Whole grain soy flour, 3 tablespoons
- Baking powder, 1 teaspoon
- 3 eggs
- Creamed cottage cheese, 1/3 cup

Method

1. In a large bowl, mix together the why protein, almond meal flour, soy flour and baking powder until well combined
2. In another bowl, whisk up the eggs and add the cottage cheese
3. Over a medium heat, heat a griddle pan and add canola oil or butter to grease
4. Drop the batter into the pan, around ¼ cup for each one
5. The batter will bubble up and this is when you should turn the pancake over and cook until it is firm to touch
6. Repeat the process until the batter is gone

Tips & Tricks/Did You Know?

You can make this recipe even more delicious by serving it with pancake syrup, the sugar free variety, or you can add toasted almonds – be careful of the extra carb content however, and add this into your consideration.

Blue Cheese and Bacon Soup

Cooking time: 35 minutes
Recipe makes 6 servings
Total carbs per serving 5.9g

Ingredients

- Bacon, 6 medium slices
- Unsalted butter, 3 tablespoons
- 2 leeks

- Mushrooms, 2 cups
- Cauliflower, 1.5 cups
- Chicken broth, 2 x 14.5oz cans
- Water, 0.5 cup
- Blue cheese, 2.5oz

Method

1. Cut the bacon into small strips
2. Cook the bacon by frying over a medium to high heat on a skillet pan, make sure they are crispy
3. Pat the bacon dry by placing on kitchen roll paper and blotting
4. Wait until the bacon is cool and then crumble it up
5. In a large pot, melt the button over a medium heat
6. Into the pot add the mushrooms and cauliflower, cook for 5 minutes and stir from time to time
7. Add the chicken, broth, and water to the pan
8. Lower the heat and simmer for 10 minutes
9. Puree the soup using a blender or a food processor in batches
10. Add each batch of soup back into the pot
11. Add the cheese into the last batch before pureeing
12. Re-heat if needed
13. Crumble the bacon over the top before serving

Tips & Tricks/Did You Know?

If you're not a fan of blue cheese, you can add Roquefort as an alternative.

Spiced Pork With Garlic Greens

Cooking time: 1 hour
Recipe makes 4 servings
Total carbs per serving 10g

Ingredients

- Olive oil, 2 tablespoons
- Red bell pepper, half, chopped
- Minced garlic, 6 cloves
- Greens, this can be frozen, and two different types at 10oz each
- Water, 1 cup
- Cider vinegar, 2 tablespoons
- Salt, ¼ teaspoon
- Pork tenderloin, 1lb, cut finely
- 2 Serrano peppers chopped finely
- Black pepper, 1 teaspoon

Method

1. On a medium heat, warm up 2 tablespoons of oil
2. Add the pepper and garlic into the pan and cook until slightly brown
3. Chop the greens
4. Add the greens and the water to the pan and allow it to boil before reducing the heat and covering the pan
5. Simmer for 20 minutes, remember to stir occasionally
6. Add the vinegar and stir, add the salt and stir
7. Remove the skillet from the heat

8. In a bowl, mix up the pork strips, red peppers, and black pepper
9. Heat another 1 tablespoon of oil in a separate skillet
10. Add the pork and cook until thoroughly heated, around 3-5 minutes
11. Serve the pork over the greens

Tips & Tricks/Did You Know?

If you don't like the heat of a serrano pepper, you can substitute this with a regular red pepper, however go for the brightest possible, to get the best amount of antioxidants into your diet. If you are using serrano peppers, do remember that you should be wearing rubber gloves when handling them, and certainly don't forget to wash your hands afterward!

Blueberry Cucumber Chiller

Cooking time: 10 minutes
Recipe makes 1 servings
Total carbs per serving 5.3g

Ingredients

- Chopped cucumber, 0.5 cup
- Lemon juice, 2 tablespoons
- Blueberries, 1 oz
- Sweetener, 0.5 teaspoons
- Rosemary, 1 teaspoon
- Ice cubes, x4

- Club soda, 4 oz

Method

1. Chop up the cucumber
2. Blend 0.5 cup of the cucumber
3. Add the lemon juice, blueberries and sugar substitute
4. Blend together thoroughly
5. Add the rosemary into the mixture and pulse the blender a couple of times
6. Strain the mixture out thoroughly
7. You can throw away the pulp
8. Into the glass place the ice, and then add the club soda (and gin if required)
9. Stir and enjoy!

Tips & Tricks/Did You Know?

You can make this particular drink alcoholic if you want to, by adding 1 fluid oz of gin into the mixture and knocking off 1 oz of club soda.

Bok Choy and Green Onions

Cooking time: 15 minutes
Recipe makes 4 servings
Total carbs per serving 3.3g

Ingredients

- Spring onions or scallions, x 4

- Tap water, 1 fluid oz
- Sugar substitute, 1 teaspoon
- Canola vegetable oil, 1 tablespoon
- Sesame oil, 1 teaspoon
- Chinese cabbage, either Bok-Choy or Pak-Choi works well, 8 heads
- Garlic, 1.5 teaspoons
- Red pepper, crushed, 1/8 teaspoons
- Peanuts in the shell, 1 cup
- Tamari soybean sauce, 2 tablespoons

Method

1. Take a small bowl and combine together the tamari, water, and sugar substitute
2. Heat up a wok or skillet pan with the canola and sesame oils
3. When the pan is hot, add in the Chinese cabbage, garlic, soy sauce and pepper
4. Stir fry for around 3 minutes
5. Stir in the peanuts to serve

Tips & Tricks/Did You Know?

Chinese cabbage has a distinct taste which certainly has the oriental about it. This recipe is not at all tasteless as the name would perhaps suggest, and it certainly goes very well on its own; having said that, if you add in the extra carbs, why not throw in some chicken and give yourself a real feast?

Baked Quesadillas

Cooking time: 20 minutes
Recipe makes 4 servings
Total carbs per serving 5.1g

Ingredients

- Light olive oil, 2 tablespoons
- Chopped onions, 2 tablespoons
- Pork chops, 16oz
- Monterey Jack cheese, 1oz
- Salsa verde, 0.25 cup
- Jalapeno pepper, x 1
- Coriander, 0.25 cup
- Black pepper, 1 teaspoon
- Salt 0.25 teaspoon
- Low carb tortilla x 1

Method

1. Preheat the oven to 230°C
2. Heat 1 tablespoon of oil in a large pan
3. Add the chopped onion and cook for 5 minutes
4. Add the onion to a bowl and add the pork, cheese, salsa, jalapeno, cilantro, pepper, and salt
5. Mix up the mixture well
6. Take the tortilla and brush one side with the rest of the oil
7. Smooth some of the mixture over the side of the tortilla that hasn't been oiled
8. Fold in half
9. Bake in the oven for 5 minutes, until golden and crisp

Tips & Tricks/Did You Know?

This particular dish is ideal for phase 2, but make sure you check the label of the tortillas, to make sure they don't contain more than 3g of carbs each. You can serve these delicious quesadillas, with sour cream if you like.

4

Recipes For The Atkins Diet
Phase 3

Quick Reminder of Phase 3

By the end of this particular phase, you will have reached that magic number, i.e. your weight loss goal. You can probably guess that in phase 3 you further increase your carbohydrate intake, again in a slow manner, by adding in extra foods from the allowance list. If you find that the scales begin to move upwards, you can go back to phase 2 again for a little longer - this is all about monitoring.

- You can eat 35g of carbohydrates per day, but you can move up to 30g and then 35g if you want to keep a handle on it a little more
- Remember to keep your protein up to the normal amount you are allowed
- You should stay in this phase until you have maintained your goal for a month without

fluctuating, but again, only weigh yourself once per week

Breakfast Mexi Peppers

Cooking time: 1 hour
Recipe makes 4 servings
Total carbs per serving 5.3g

Ingredients

- Pork and beef chorizo, 4oz
- Ground beef, 4 oz
- Chopped onions, 0.5 cup
- Shredded cheddar cheese, 0.25 cup
- 3 legs
- Sweet red peppers, x 2

Method

1. Preheat the oven to 200°C
2. Line a baking tray with foil
3. Cook the chorizo until brown, make sure you drain off the fat
4. Into a small mixing bowl combine the chorizo and ground beef
5. Add in the onion, cheese, and eggs
6. Cut the peppers in half and remove the seeds
7. Fill each of the peppers with the mixture
8. Bake in the oven for half an hour

Tips & Tricks/Did You Know?

This morning snack is certainly going to keep you full until lunchtime, as it is packed with 21.3g of protein, meaning you're not likely to feel hungry or want to snack mid-morning. Again, go for the reddest pepper you can find, as this will have more vitamins.

Burgundy Chicken

Cooking time: 15 minutes
Recipe makes 4 servings
Total carbs per serving 3.5g

Ingredients

- Celery, 1 medium
- Extra virgin olive oil, 2 tablespoons
- Half a medium carrot
- Garlic, 1 teaspoon
- Parsley, 2 tablespoons
- Chicken broth, 0.5 cup
- Red wine, 4 fluid oz
- Cooked chicken thighs, boneless, 32oz
- 1 onion
- Bay leaf, 0.5 teaspoon, crumbled
- Cooked ham, fresh, boneless, 2oz

Method

1. Over a medium heat, add oil to a large skillet
2. Add the onion, carrot and celery, cooking until soft
3. Add the ham and garlic, cooking for a further 2 minutes

4. Add the mixture to a separate bowl
5. Cook the chicken thighs on all sides until brown
6. Add the wine, broth, and bay leaf to the pan and reduce the heat down to medium
7. Cook for half an hour, until the chicken is cooked and liquid is reduced
8. Add the vegetables and ham back into the pan
9. Mix everything up and heat for a further 5 minutes

Tips & Tricks/Did You Know?

Red table wine works best for this particular recipe, and this also doesn't need to be the most expensive brand to add taste. You can also make this recipe in phase 1, if you take out the carrot.

Almond & Pineapple Smoothie

Cooking time: 5 minutes
Recipe makes 1 servings
Total carbs per serving 17g

Ingredients

- Plain yogurt, 0.5 cup
- Pineapple, 2.5 oz
- Whole almonds, x 20
- Pure almond milk, 0.5 cup

Method

1. Place all ingredients into a blender

2. Combine until smooth
3. Serve immediately

Tips & Tricks/Did You Know?

This particular drink is very high in carbs, so it should be kept into moderation and only consumed occasionally. Phase 3 introduces more in the way of exotic fruits, but pineapple does have many weight loss busting elements, so make sure you have this occasionally, however only ever use fresh, canned is not as good.

Beef Saute With Vegetables and Romaine

Cooking time: 45 minutes
Recipe makes 6 servings
Total carbs per serving 6.3g

Ingredients

- Ground beef, 1.5lbs
- Chopped onions, 0.25 cup
- Green pepper (sweeter the better), chopped, 0.25 cup
- Canned tomato sauce, 15oz
- Tomato paste, 4 tablespoons
- Sugar substitute, 3 teaspoons
- Shredded Romaine lettuce, 6 cups
- Cheddar cheese, 6oz

Method

- Over a medium to high heat, brown the beef
- Add the onions and peppers towards the end of the beef cooking
- Add the tomato sauce, tomato paste, and sugar substitute, salt, and pepper
- Turn the heat down to low and simmer for around half an hour
- Once cooked, serve straight away over Romaine with cheddar sprinkled on top

Tips & Tricks/Did You Know?

You can mix this recipe up and make it a more Mexican style by adding cayenne pepper to the beef, and you could even use it in wraps for a tortilla-style; just remember to add the extra carbs for the wrap.

Buffalo Chicken Wings

Cooking time: 45 minutes
Recipe makes 6 servings
Total carbs per serving 1.9g

Ingredients

- Cider vinegar, 1 cup
- Canola vegetable oil, 0.5 cup
- Black pepper, 0.5 teaspoon
- Garlic powder, 0.5 teaspoon
- Salt, 1 teaspoon
- Celery salt, 0.25 teaspoon
- Cayenne pepper, 1/8 teaspoon

- Chicken wings, 32oz
- 1 egg
- Mayonnaise, 1 cup
- Sour cream, 0.5 cup
- Spring onions or 1 scallion
- Blue cheese, 1/3 cup
- Lemon juice, 0.5 fluid oz

Method

1. Preheat the oven to 230°C
2. Into a medium bowl, beat the egg and add vinegar, salt, oil, pepper, garlic powder, celery salt, and cayenne. Stir well
3. Dip the chicken into the marinade and place on a baking tray
4. Bake in the oven for half an hour, turning regularly
5. You may need to re-brush with the marinade occasionally
6. Cook until the wings are crispy and cooked through
7. Into another bowl, mix the mayonnaise, sour cream, cheese, scallion/spring onion, lemon juice, and garlic
8. Serve the chicken whilst hot with the dipping sauce in a separate pot

Tips & Tricks/Did You Know?

If cayenne pepper is a little too spicy for you, you can replace this with a milder red pepper, and if you don't like blue cheese, replace it with Roquefort, for a creamier taste to this classic dish.

Baked Brie with Sun-Dried Tomatoes and Pine Nuts

Cooking time: 15 minutes
Recipe makes 6 servings
Total carbs per serving 0.5g

Ingredients

- Brie cheese, 8oz
- Chopped sun-dried tomatoes, 1 tablespoon
- Parsley, 1 tablespoon
- Dried pine nuts, 0.5 oz

Method

1. Preheat the oven to 230°C
2. Trim the cheese to get rid of any rind
3. Find a pie plate or something alternative and place the cheese inside
4. In a bowl combine the sun-dried tomatoes and the parsley
5. Spread the mixture over the cheese evenly
6. Sprinkle the pine nuts over the top
7. Place in the oven for 10 minutes

Tips & Tricks/Did You Know?

This dish is a fantastic party food suggestion as well as a meal or snack in itself – almost like a fondue, you can add dipping aids, such as low carb bread or tortillas, provided you factor in the extra carbs for your daily intake.

Grilled Tofu With Peanut Sauce

Cooking time: 30 minutes
Recipe makes 4 servings
Total carbs per serving 10g

Ingredients

- 2 x tofu packages, 14 oz
- Canola oil, 2 tablespoons for tofu, and 3 tablespoons for sauce
- Salt, 0.25 teaspoons
- Ground black pepper, 0.25 teaspoons
- Tamarind paste, 1 tablespoon
- Minced garlic, 1 tablespoon
- Minced shallot, 1 tablespoon
- Chili paste, 1 teaspoon
- Chopped peanuts, 0.25 cup
- Peanut butter, 2 tablespoons
- Unsweetened coconut milk, 1/3 cup
- Cilantro, chopped, 2 tablespoons

Method

1. Take each tofu pack and cut each into four blocks
2. Take 2 tablespoons of canola oil and rub the tofu with it, add salt and pepper to season
3. Add the tamarind paste into 1/3 cup of water and dissolve
4. Heat 3 tablespoons of canola oil
5. Add the garlic and shallots to the pan, cooked for 1 minute

6. Add the chili paste and peanuts, stir constantly
7. Add the peanut butter and dissolved tamarind, then the coconut milk
8. Cover the mixture and keep warm
9. Preheat the grill on a low temperature
10. Grill the tofu for 10 seconds on each side
11. Serve by pouring the sauce over each block of tofu, and sprinkle with cilantro

Tips & Tricks/Did You Know?

Smooth peanut butter works best for this recipe, however if you are struggling to find it, or you prefer a different variety you can add this, simply add the extra carb intake (if any) to the total.

Brisket With Mushrooms

Cooking time: 135 minutes
Recipe makes 10 servings
Total carbs per serving 2.4g

Ingredients

- Dried Porcini mushrooms, 15 pieces
- Extra virgin olive oil, 1 tablespoon
- Beef brisket, 4lb
- Onion x 2
- Garlic, 1.5 teaspoons
- Beef broth, 1 can/14oz
- Crumbled Bay leaf, 1 teaspoon
- Salt, 0.5 teaspoon

- Black pepper, 0.25 teaspoon

Method

1. Into a small bowl add the mushrooms and 0.75 cups of water
2. Microwave the mixture on high until the water is boiling
3. Allow to cool
4. Over a medium heat, warm up the oil
5. Take the brisket and warm it on one side, turn over and add the onions
6. Add the garlic when the onions are brown, cook for a further one minute
7. Take the mushrooms from the liquid (keep the liquid to one side)
8. Rinse the mushrooms and chop roughly
9. Place the mushrooms to the brisket
10. Strain the reserved liquid from the mushrooms and add to the brisket mixture
11. Add the broth, Bay leaf, salt and pepper
12. Cover the mixture and reduce the heat down to low
13. Cook for 2-2.5 hours and then remove the brisket
14. Turn the heat up and cook until the juices are thickened
15. Cut the brisket into slices and serve with the liquid mixture

Tips & Tricks/Did You Know?

If you're looking for a winter warmer, this dish works fantastic as an alternative to old fashioned stews. You will also get a huge hit of protein too, which we know is very important on the Atkins diet, no matter what stage you are in.

Spicy Hummus

Cooking time: 15 minutes
Recipe makes 16 servings
Total carbs per serving 11g

Ingredients

- Chickpeas, 2 cups (drained and rinsed)
- Lime juice, 6 tablespoons
- Extra virgin olive oil, 0.25 cup
- Sesame paste, 0.25 cup
- Roasted red pepper in a jar, x1
- Minced garlic, 2 cloves
- Ground cumin, 2 teaspoons
- Salt, 1 teaspoon
- Cayenne pepper, 0.5 teaspoon
- Water, 0.5 cup

Method

1. Place the chickpeas, lime juice, olive oil, sesame paste, red pepper, garlic, cumin, salt, and cayenne into a food processor until it forms a smooth paste in consistency
2. Whilst you are pureeing, pour the water very slowly into the tube until it is as thick or thin as you like
3. Serve or store

Tips & Tricks/Did You Know?

Although you can easily buy hummus in the supermarket, it can be quite expensive, so it is much more cost effective, and probably healthier to make your own. If you want to give your hummus a spicy kick, simply add more cayenne pepper. You can store this recipe for up to 2 days in the fridge.

Caramelised Pear Custard

Cooking time: 10 minutes
Recipe makes 8 servings
Total carbs per serving 7.6g

Ingredients

- Butter, 2 tablespoons
- Xylitol, 2 tablespoons
- Ground cardamom, 0.25 teaspoon
- Pears, x 2
- 3 eggs
- 2 egg yolks
- Heavy cream, 2 cups
- Low calorie maple syrup (sugar free) 1/8 cups
- Rum, 0.5 fluid oz
- Vanilla extract, 1 teaspoon

Method

1. Preheat the oven to 190°C

2. Warm up the butter, xylitol, and the cardamom over a medium to high heat
3. Slice up the pears into wedges, around 0.5" each
4. Add the pears once the butter is melted and leave for 4 minutes on each side
5. Place the pears into a casserole dish or high sided plate
6. Pour 2 tablespoons of the maple syrup over the pears
7. Into a small bowl, mix up the eggs, yolks, heavy cream, syrup, rum, and vanilla
8. Pour over the pears
9. Bake in the oven for around 20 minutes
10. Brush the top of the dish with the rest of the syrup

Tips & Tricks/Did You Know?

You can omit the rum if you want to go for a non-alcoholic option to this dish.

Cheese Baked Eggs

Cooking time: 30 minutes
Recipe makes 4 servings
Total carbs per serving 10g

Ingredients

- Unsalted butter, 1 teaspoon
- 2 eggs
- Heavy cream, 2 tablespoons
- Grated parmesan cheese, 2 tablespoons

Method

1. Preheat the oven to 190°C
2. Find an oven safe dish and melt the butter, coating the inside of the dish
3. Into a small bowl, mix together the eggs and cream
4. Add the cheese, ground black pepper, and salt, mix together
5. Bake in the oven for 10 minutes

Tips & Tricks/Did You Know?

This particular dish is actually suitable for all phases, but is a delicious recipe to try in phase 3, if you are running low on your carb intake for that particular meal. You could of course add low carb bread if you have a few extra carbs spare.

Barbecue Sauce

Cooking time: 25 minutes
Recipe makes 10 servings
Total carbs per serving 3.7g

Ingredients

- Extra virgin olive oil, 1 tablespoon
- Chopped onions, 0.25 cup
- Tomato paste, 2 tablespoons
- Chili powder, 1 teaspoon
- Cumin, 1 teaspoon
- Garlic powder, 0.75 teaspoon

- Yellow mustard seed, 0.75 teaspoon
- Ground allspice, 0.75 teaspoon
- Cayenne pepper, 1/8 teaspoon
- Ketchup, unsweetened, 1.5 cups
- Cider vinegar, 1 tablespoon
- Worcestershire sauce, 2/3 tablespoons
- Sugar substitute, 2 tablespoons
- Instant dry coffee powder, 0.25 teaspoons

Method

1. Over a medium to high heat, warm up the oil
2. Add the onion and cook for around 3 minutes
3. Add the tomato paste, chili, cumin, garlic, mustard, allspice, cayenne pepper and cook for another minute
4. Add the ketchup, vinegar, Worcestershire sauce, sugar substitute, and coffee
5. Simmer the mixture and stir occasionally for around 8 minutes – it should thicken up considerably
6. Serve or wait to cool before storing

Tips & Tricks/Did You Know?

Each particular serving of this sauce works out at a generous 2 tablespoons, which works out your total carb intake for this recipe. If you go over, remember to adjust accordingly; it's very easy to have too much sauce!

Recipes For The Atkins Diet
Phase 4

Quick Reminder of Phase 4

Phase 4 is your maintenance phase, and this is where you are going to stay for the rest of your life. Don't panic, it's not as drastic as it sounds! Basically, at this point you are at your goal and you have now recognized your carb intake level, the natural amount you can eat without the scales budging either way. If you do find you are putting weight on, you can drop back down a phase, or even go back to phase 1 if you need to – the Atkins Diet is personal in that way.

- Stick to your personal carb intake level
- Remember to keep your protein up
- Mix and match your food to stop boredom creeping in
- Try and recognize this as a healthy lifestyle, rather than a dietary phase

Asparagus and Leek Soup

Cooking time: 30 minutes
Recipe makes 4 servings
Total carbs per serving 5.2g

Ingredients

- Unsalted butter, 2 tablespoons
- Leek x 1
- Asparagus, 0.75lb
- Garlic, 1 teaspoon
- Chicken broth, 14.5oz
- Heavy cream, 1/3 cup

Method

1. In a large pot, melt the butter, before adding the leeks and cooking for around 3 minutes
2. Add the asparagus and cook for a further minute
3. Add the garlic and cook for half a minute
4. Add the broth and bring the pot to the boil
5. Turn the heat down and simmer for around 10 minutes
6. Add the cream, salt and the pepper
7. Blend the soup in a blender or food processor
8. Heat up if required
9. Season to taste

Tips & Tricks/Did You Know?

You can make this soup in batches and keep for a few days,

provided you wait for it to cool completely and then store in an airtight container, in the fridge.

Chocolate and Hazelnut Mousse

Cooking time: 3.5 hours
Recipe makes 6 servings
Total carbs per serving 3g

Ingredients

- Low carb chocolate, 4oz
- Unsalted butter, 4 teaspoons
- Hazelnut syrup (sugar free), 4 teaspoons
- Heavy cream, 1 1/3 cups
- Sugar substitute, 4 teaspoons
- Chopped and toasted hazelnuts, 4 tablespoons
- Fresh raspberries, x6

Method

1. Into a small bowl melt the chocolate, the butter, and the syrup over a low heat
2. Transfer into a bowl and set to one side
3. Add the cream and sugar substitute into another bowl and whip together well
4. Fold 1/3 of the mixture into the chocolate and stir
5. Combine the rest and stir
6. Add in the hazelnuts and raspberry as a garnish

Tips & Tricks/Did You Know?

This particular delicious treat will keep for up to 3 hours, but transfer to the fridge if you aren't eating straight away.

Crispy, Spicy Cauliflower

Cooking time: 30 minutes
Recipe makes 4 servings
Total carbs per serving 5g

Ingredients

- 2 eggs
- Cauliflower florets, 4 cups
- Almond flour, 4 tablespoons
- Chili powder, 1 teaspoon
- Canola oil
- Fish sauce, 2 teaspoons
- Lime juice, 1 tablespoon
- Scallions, chopped, 1 tablespoon

Method

1. Combine the eggs into a large bowl and toss in the cauliflower florets, coating completely
2. Place the florets onto a plate
3. Add the almond flour and chili powder, sprinkling over the top
4. Using a wok or high sided frying pan, fill with canola oil and heat to 170°C
5. Fry the florets in the oil
6. Transfer to paper towels to absorb extra oil
7. Drizzle with fish sauce and lime juice

8. Add the chopped scallions as a garnish

Tips & Tricks/Did You Know?

If you're not the biggest cauliflower fan, you can deep fry other vegetables, simply being careful of the carb amount and adjusting the number accordingly. Having said that, cauliflower does give you a big 7g of protein.

Asian Vegetable Bowl

Cooking time: 20 minutes
Recipe makes 6 servings
Total carbs per serving 4.6g

Ingredients

- Spring onions, 3 cups
- Mushrooms, 2 cups
- Tamari soybean sauce, 4 tablespoons
- Ginger, 3 teaspoons
- Garlic, 1 clove
- Serrano pepper, x1
- Sliced red tomato, 1 cup
- Tofu, the firm variety, 6oz
- Carrot
- Cilantro, 0.5oz
- Chinese cabbage, shredded, 2 cups
- Chicken broth, 6 cups

Method

1. Heat up the broth and tamari and bring to the boil
2. Turn down the heat and add the Chinese cabbage, mushrooms, ginger, garlic, and chili
3. Simmer for around 5 minutes
4. Add the tomatoes, onions, tofu, and carrot, cook for around 1 minute more
5. Stir in the cilantro and serve

Tips & Tricks/Did You Know?

You can make this particular recipe acceptable for phase 1 if you simply take out the carrot. If you are vegetarian, then simply omit the chicken broth and replace it with the vegetable variety.

Banana & Coconut Rum

Cooking time: 5 minutes
Recipe makes 1 servings
Total carbs per serving 8.9g

Ingredients

- Small banana, 1/3
- Coconut cream, 1/3 cup
- Rum, 1 fluid oz
- Ice cubes, x2
- Sweetener, 0.75 teaspoon

Method

1. Combine the banana, coconut, rum, and sugar substitute into a blender, before adding the ice
2. Blend until totally combined
3. Serve in a glass – delicious!

Tips & Tricks/Did You Know?

You can go for spiced rum if you prefer but do check regarding the carb intake of your particular chosen variety – some do harbor hidden carbs! If you want to go non-alcoholic, simply use rum extract rather than actual rum.

Breakfast Sausage Sauteed with Red & Green Peppers

Cooking time: 15 minutes
Recipe makes 1 servings
Total carbs per serving 3g

Ingredients

- Canola oil, 1 teaspoon
- Turkey breakfast sausage, 4 links (cooked)
- Red sweet pepper, 1 quarter
- Green sweet pepper, 1 quarter
- Monterey Jack cheese, 1oz

Method

1. Over a medium to high heat, add the oil to a skillet pan and heat up
2. You can either crumble the sausage or slice after

cooking, but add to the pan and brown for around
3 minutes

3. Add the red and green peppers
4. Cook for a further 5 minutes
5. Sprinkle on the cheese, allowing to melt
6. Serve

Tips & Tricks/Did You Know?

Different types of breakfast sausage work just as well if you
don't like turkey, but do check the carb intake amount.

Cajun Pork Chops

Cooking time: 20 minutes
Recipe makes 4 servings
Total carbs per serving 0.7g

Ingredients

- Paprika, 1 tablespoon
- Cumin, 0.5 teaspoon
- Ground sage, 0.5 teaspoon
- Black pepper, 0.5 teaspoon
- Garlic powder, 0.5 teaspoon
- Cayenne pepper, 0.5 teaspoon
- Pork chops, 24oz
- Unsalted butter, 0.5 tablespoons
- Canola oil, 0.5 tablespoons

Method

1. Into a bowl, combine all the spices onto a plate
2. Season the pork chops onto both sides
3. On a high heat, melt the butter and oil
4. Cook the chops in the skillet on a medium heat for just under 10 minutes, turn halfway through
5. Serve

Tips & Tricks/Did You Know?

If you are running low on carbs on a particular day and you want a hearty, delicious meal, this is a great option, which is extremely low in carb intake, whilst being high in protein.

Breakfast Burrito

Cooking time: 20 minutes
Recipe makes 2 servings
Total carbs per serving 7.9g

Ingredients

- Salt, 0.5 teaspoon
- Cayenne pepper, 0.25 teaspoon
- Canola oil, 1 tablespoon
- Eggs x 4
- Sweet red peppers, 3 tablespoons
- Spring onions, 2 tablespoons
- Jalapeno pepper, x1
- Low carb tortillas, x2
- Tabasco sauce, 1/8 teaspoon
- Salsa, 2oz

Method

1. Whisk up the eggs, cayenne, and salt
2. Over a medium heat, toast the tortillas for a minute, turning and repeating
3. Cook the oil, red pepper, spring onion, and jalapeno until soft, for about 3 minutes
4. Add the eggs and stir, cooking for around 2 minutes more
5. Divide the mixture between the tortillas
6. Season with the tabasco sauce
7. Roll up the tortillas
8. Serve with the salsa and greens

Tips & Tricks/Did You Know?

Be careful of the brand of salsa you use, and always check the label. Every single company makes their product differently and some may have a higher carb content than others – shop around.

Key Lime Mousse

Cooking time: 1 hour 20 minutes
Recipe makes 4 servings
Total carbs per serving 4g

Ingredients

- Mashed avocados, 2 cups
- Lime zest, 0.5 teaspoon
- Lime juice, 3 oz

- Powdered xylitol, 0.25 cups
- Stevia crystals, 0.5 teaspoon
- Vanilla extract, 2 teaspoons
- Salt, 1 pinch
- Ground cinnamon, 1 pinch
- Ground nutmeg, 1 pinch
- Almond butter, 2 tablespoons
- Extract (your choice), 0.25 teaspoons
- Strawberries, 0.25 cup

Method

1. Into a food processor, place all ingredients (except strawberries) and combine until creamy
2. Remove from the processor and allow it to rest for around 20 minutes at the very least
3. Add the strawberries as a garnish

Tips & Tricks/Did You Know?

For the best taste, make sure you go for medium ripe avocados; if they are too ripe the taste will be too strong, and if they are under ripe, the taste will be neither here nor there.

Cauliflower Potato Salad

Cooking time: 20 minutes
Recipe makes 6 servings
Total carbs per serving 3.8g

Ingredients

- Spring onions, x 3
- Mayonnaise, 4 tablespoons
- Lemon juice, 1 fluid oz
- Sugar substitute, 1 teaspoon
- Ground mustard, 0.5 teaspoon
- Cauliflower head x 1
- Jalapeno pepper x1
- Salt, 1/8 teaspoon
- Black pepper, 1/8 teaspoon

Method

1. Cook the cauliflower first of all in salted water, to your taste
2. Drain and pat dry the cauliflower
3. Mix together the mayonnaise, lemon juice, sugar substitute, and the mustard, until well combined
4. Add the cauliflower, pepper, and onion
5. Mix together until well coated
6. Add salt and pepper

Tips & Tricks/Did You Know?

For the best flavor, place the dish into the fridge after mixing together and leave for at least half an hour.

Greek Salad

Cooking time: 20 minutes
Recipe makes 6 servings
Total carbs per serving 5g

Ingredients

- Feta cheese, cut into chunks, 150g
- Feta brine, 2 tablespoon
- Fresh lime juice, 3 tablespoons
- Extra virgin olive oil, 4 tablespoons
- Plum tomatoes, 1 cup
- Cucumber, 0.75 cup
- Red onion, 0.5 cup
- Green bell pepper, 0.75 cup
- Black olives, 1/3 cup
- Arugula, 2 cups
- Dried oregano, 2 tablespoons
- Salt, 1 teaspoon

Method

1. Blend up half of the feta cheese, brine, olive oil, and lemon juice in a blender or food processor
2. Mix together the rest of the ingredients into a bowl (except the arugula)
3. Add the dressing and mix
4. Add the arugula and toss gently

Tips & Tricks/Did You Know?

This particular salad works well as a side salad to a main meal, as it is low in carbs and not the highest in protein either – add a meat dish to up your protein amount.

Cheese Sauce

Cooking time: 15 minutes
Recipe makes 8 servings
Total carbs per serving 1.5g

Ingredients

- Heavy cream, 1 cup
- Roquefort cheese, 0.5 cup (crumbled)
- Jarlsberg cheese, 2oz
- Grated parmesan cheese, 0.25 cup
- Paprika, 0.5 teaspoon

Method

1. Over a low heat, heat up the cream
2. Add in the Roquefort until melted
3. Add in the Jarlsberg until melted
4. Add in the parmesan until melted
5. Add the paprika and continue to cook until hot and smooth, stirring regularly
6. Season with salt and pepper

Tips & Tricks/Did You Know?

If you don't like any of the cheese in this particular recipe, you can substitute them for others, but simply check if there are any additional carbs to take into account for your calculations.

Afterword

This book is designed to give you inspiration and ideas for what you can eat during your time on the Atkins Diet, at each phase. Probably the most daunting thing about starting a diet is 'what am I going to eat?' and worrying about what you are going to miss. The main plus point of the Atkins Diet, aside from the weight loss side of things, is that you can eat many things that you can't eat on a regular diet, and because of that you don't get hungry, and you're not at the mercy of cravings.

For this reason alone, the Atkins Diet is very easy to follow.

If you try even half of the recipes we have talked about in this book, you will see how delicious the Atkins Diet can be, and you will certainly be very full indeed as a result!

Of course, you can modify any of our recipes, provided you take into account the amount of carbohydrates you are taking in, as well as making sure you get your protein allowance per day; this currently stands at 4-6oz per day, depending on your body weight, so check current guidelines to make sure you are getting enough – protein is extremely important.

Give these recipes a try for yourself, and see how easy and delicious the Atkins Diet can be.

www.ingramcontent.com/pod-product-compliance
Lightning Source LLC
Chambersburg PA
CBHW032103280526
45784CB00013B/3012